M000015118

Breaking the Curse
of a
Death Sentence

By Jan Christie Green

Forwarded by Dr. Rodney Derrick

Table of Contents

Forward

This book is an example of what happens when you fail to give up even in dire circumstances.

Sickle Cell Anemia is one of many diseases that comes into our lives without permission.

In *Breaking the Curse of a Death Sentence,* Jan Christie Green teaches you how to continue with your dreams despite of any illness or disease that you may have been diagnosed with. She provides you with practical tools and spiritual concepts to help you live life to the fullest.

As a person who battled prostate cancer, I know how it is to live in uncertainty and not know what will happen from day to day. Living with illness and disease can cause you to walk in constant fear. Yet, I found this book as a great resource that inspired me to live my best life despite of the unknown.

Jan, thank you so much for this lifeline to so many of us that are dealing with things that caught us by surprise.

Breaking the Curse of a Death Sentence will make a difference in your life. The words in this book will help you to take back your life despite of pain.

As you read this book, I encourage you to see it as opening a gift. With each page, you will unwrap healing, inspiration, and the tools needed to rise above any dire situation that has tried to prevent you from living your best life. Ultimately, you will unwrap the stamina that you need to survive.

Dr. Rodney Derrick

Senior Pastor Life Community Church, SA

San Antonio, TX

This book is dedicated to my loving sister, Billie Joyce Young, who passed away at the tender age of 15 from the many complications of Sickle Cell Anemia.

Introduction

This book gives practical and spiritual concepts to help those who suffer from the devastating effects of incurable diseases, such as Sickle Cell Anemia and Cancer.

Healing begins in the mind and resonates throughout the body.

To walk in healing, a person must educate themselves about the illness that is negatively impacting their bodies, be willing and able to speak positive affirmations to their body, and change every day habits to improve health, such as what they eat and how they think.

Faith is a necessary tool that must be practiced daily if one is to see healing manifest.

"And they overcame… by the blood of the lamb and by the word of their testimony" *(Rev.12:11).*

From as far back as I can remember, I was a victim of Sickle Cell Anemia. I was a twin and the middle child of six. My twin brother passed away at birth. My parents were not aware that they were both carriers of the Sickle Cell trait until I was born and started having major health issues. Blood test came back positive for the full-blown disease. One of the things I will never forget is the many times I was rushed to the hospital because I could not stop coughing up blood clots and the excruciating pain that I suffered in my arms and legs. Throughout the first 24 years of my life, I received tons of blood transfusions, suffered through collapsed lungs, jaundice, pneumonia, meningitis, and the pain that often caused swelling in my joints. This disease robbed me of the ability to successfully carry my first two babies causing me to miscarry them only weeks after impregnation.

However, through this storm, Yahweh[1] came through for me in that He brought healing to my body and caused my misery to become my ministry. Now at the age of 47, I am no longer a victim of Sickle Cell Anemia, but I am an overcomer. I have not had a Sickle Cell crisis since the age of 24 and I am the mother of two beautiful young ladies.

I write this book to encourage you that what Yahweh has done for me, He will surely do for you if you believe.

It is by your faith that you shall walk in healing.

---

[1] Yahweh – Hebrew name for the one true God, creator of the Universe.

Know that true deliverance is granted for you to walk out your divine purpose.

In this book you will find many testimonies that I will share with you from my own life experiences. You will find practical methods that Yahweh gave to me to overcome the devastating effects of the disease and you will find the tools you need to *Breaking the Curse of a Death Sentence.*

When the doctors said I would die, it was Yahweh who said, "*You shall not die but live and declare the works of the Lord.*[2]

It is my prayer that as you read this book and apply its truths and principals that you will find that Yahweh is ready to meet your need, heal your body, and strengthen you to walk out the plans that He has ordained for your life. They

---

[2] Psalms 118:17

are plans of peace and not of evil to give you an expected end.[3]

---

[3] Jeremiah 29:11

The Curse

evil or misfortune that comes as if in answer to someone's request

As a victim of Sickle Cell Anemia, I felt as though I was cursed. Every time I turned around, I was under its influence. I could not escape its devastating effects. One moment I was fine, and the next moment I was in excruciating pain as though some unseen force hated me and used me as a pin cushion whenever it was irritated with me. It did not matter where I was or what I was doing, this curse of sickness invaded my agenda whenever it pleased and without my permission. I felt it was not fair. While my siblings played and enjoyed their youth, I was either at home taking pain meds or in the hospital fighting for my very life. I was accursed for sure and there was nothing that my loved ones could do to free me.

The definition of a curse is the pronouncement of evil or misfortune that is inflicted or wished upon another at the heartfelt invoking or calling down of that person's enemy.[4] A curse was considered to possess the authority to carry out the antagonistic impact that it was sent to do. When we look at the impact of a curse in the Bible, we first see it mentioned in Genesis chapter 3. It tells of the event where Yahweh confronts the serpent for beguiling Eve into disobeying Him by eating of the tree of the knowledge of good and evil. Yahweh looked at the serpent and said, *"Because thou hast done this, thou art cursed above all cattle, and above every beast of the field; upon thy belly shalt thou go, and dust shalt thou eat all the days of thy life: And I will put enmity between thee and the woman, and between thy seed and her seed; it shall bruise thy head, and thou shalt bruise his heel."*

Next, Yahweh turned to humanity and said *"Unto the woman…, I will greatly multiply thy sorrow and thy*

---

[4] https://en.oxforddictionaries.com/definition/curse

conception; in sorrow thou shalt bring forth children; and thy desire shall be to thy husband, and he shall rule over thee. And unto Adam he said, Because thou hast hearkened unto the voice of thy wife, and hast eaten of the tree, of which I commanded thee, saying, Thou shalt not eat of it: cursed is the ground for thy sake; in sorrow shalt thou eat of it all the days of thy life; Thorns also and thistles shall it bring forth to thee; and thou shalt eat the herb of the field; In the sweat of thy face shalt thou eat bread, till thou return unto the ground; for out of it wast thou taken: for dust thou art, and unto dust shalt thou return.[5]

In these scripture passages, we see that a curse was initially placed on the serpent whose motivation was to bring separation between Yahweh and humanity. Mankind was Yahweh's most precious creation. We were designed to be in constant communication and

---

[5] Genesis 3:13-19

fellowship with our Creator. Satan was jealous of that relationship and came in the form of a serpent to seduce mankind into partaking of the very thing that would separate them from Yahweh, sin. Therefore, the very moment Eve took a bite of the fruit from the forbidden tree, all humanity fell into the devastating effect of sin. A curse was placed on all humanity and creation that would cause a domino effect of corruption. As part of that impact, along came all kinds of hardships, infirmities, sicknesses, and even physical and spiritual death. Prior to the fall of Adam and Eve, sin, disease, and death did not exist. It was Yahweh's intention to commune with his creation eternally. Because we are now living in a fallen world, we become subject to its fallen nature. Unfortunately, that means that we are vulnerable to illnesses that we did not ask for.

Sickle Cell Anemia, along with other curable and incurable diseases, are a part of that curse that was provoked on humanity during the days of Adam and Eve. As mentioned before, a curse is purposely placed to bring about destruction to the one it is imposed upon. So, you may be asking why is it that a God of love and compassion would want to place a curse of destruction on those whom He claims to love? The answer is found in the law of cause and effect. This law or principal states that for every action taken there is an effect, and for every effect that is created, there is a cause.[6] In Genesis 2, Yahweh told Adam that he could eat as much as he wanted of every tree in the garden, except for one. This was a limitation that Yahweh had put on his creation, mankind. It is what separated the created from the Creator.

---

[6] https://blog.iqmatrix.com/law-of-cause-effect

Yahweh said, "*But of the tree of the knowledge of good and evil, thou shalt not eat of it: for in the day that thou eatest thereof thou shalt surely die.*"

Disobedience on behalf of creation was the cause, and death was the effect. Once Adam and Eve disobeyed Yahweh and ate of that tree, it caused or produced the effect of them becoming as gods. They received knowledge of the difference between good and evil which brought about the effect or consequences of sin, causing the effect of death. As we continue to read the story, we find out that this death was not a physical death or termination of life, but it was a spiritual death or termination of fellowship between Yahweh and humanity, causing separation. Now that humanity had fallen into sin and their eyes were open to its' consequences, Yahweh could not allow for his creation to survive eternally in a fallen state.

Therefore, sin took its course to include death and destruction. The real enemy was that old serpent who knew the cause and effect and enticed Eve, the mother of all living, to be subject to it.

As a part of this fallen world, I was born into a family who had the trait of Sickle Cell Anemia in their bloodline. Both my father and mother carried the trait without knowledge. Unlike Sickle Cell Disease, Sickle Cell Trait means that a person carries one defective gene in their body that can cause the disease but is not sufficient being alone. Therefore, that person can live a normal life without any negative health impacts related to the disease. However, that person does have the ability to pass that defective gene on to their children. This is what took place in my family line. As mention before, unbeknownst to them, both my parents carried a defective gene aligned to

Sickle Cell Anemia. Out of the six children that they had, both abnormal genes were passed to two of us, my younger sister and me. As a result, we both were born with full-blown Sickle Cell Disease.

Sickle Cell Disease is a curse passed down from generation to generation. It is a disease where the person is born with two genes that causes the production of abnormal hemoglobin or the protein substance in red blood cells that is responsible for carrying oxygen to the major bodily organs.[7] People all over the world, to mainly include, but not limited to African-Americans, are impacted by Sickle Cell Trait and Sickle Cell Disease. Because of the abnormal hemoglobin, the victim's red blood cells are often distorted as sickle-shaped, instead of circle shaped, as the

---

[7] http://www.hematology.org/Patients/Anemia/Sickle-Cell-Trait.aspx

reason for the name of the disease. These sickle -cell shaped blood cells are weakened and do not last long as they easily break down and are unable to pass through the smallest blood vessel.

I must inform you that I am not a physician, but from my own life experience and the research that I have done, I can tell you that Sickle Cell Disease causes many extreme health issues that prevents the victim from living a normal life. It causes severe pain in body extremities, difficulty in breathing, and the defamation of bodily organs, such as the brain, heart, and lungs. Sadly, to say, this disease has also caused loss of life in many of its victims at young ages.

Growing up with this disease, I could not participate in sports, nor regular gym activities. There were many times that I had to sit out in gym class watching my peers merrily participate while I suffered from aches and pains in my physical body. I missed school many times due to being hospitalized because of having Sickle Cell crises.

A Sickle Cell crisis is caused by the lack of healthy hemoglobin circulating red blood cells to bodily organs. It is triggered by the breaking down of the red blood cell supply. For example, an adult without Sickle Cell normally has a red blood cell count around 4.1 to 6.2 million red blood cells per microliter.[8] The normal life cycle of their red blood cells is around 110-120 days. Unfortunately for those with Sickle Cell, the red blood cell count is much lower and its' life cycle only last about 10-20 days.[9]

If the patient's body organs are not nourished with a healthy flow of

---

[8] https://www.verywellhealth.com/red-blood-cell-rbc-count-1942659
[9] https://www.mayoclinic.org/diseases-conditions/sickle-cell-anemia/symptoms-causes/syc-20355876

blood, then it is deprived of the necessary oxygen it needs to function properly. This lack of flow is what causes pain in body parts as healthy red blood cells quickly break down and the supply of oxygen quickly diminishes.[10] The many times this happened to me, I found myself being rushed to the hospital in crisis mode that lasted from several hours to several days. I had sharp stabbing pain in my back, arms, legs, knees, and chest. Many times, I knew I was about to die because the pain was so unbearable. The only thing the doctors could do was give me temporary pain medications that knocked me out my misery. While under their influence, the doctors began an incurable treatment to help me only manage, but not heal, the dilemma. That treatment came in the form of putting IV's in the veins that they could find, whether that was in my hands, arms, or feet. Then, they would

---

[10] https://www.aafp.org/afp/2000/0301/p1363.html

pump fluids in me to help liquify any areas where clumped blood cells were found to induce a healthy blood flow. However, there were times when things were more complicated. Because of the major organs being deprived of the oxygen they needed, I became more vulnerable to other diseases or illnesses. I was quick to catch pneumonia in both lungs and there was the time as a toddler when I caught meningitis, causing some damage to my brain cells.

The routine of being in and out of the hospital became the norm for me. I could see no way out of this curse, and in my house, there were no whispers of hope. I knew of Yahshua[11] but I did not know, at this tender age, of his love for me that would cause him to have the desire and the ability to

---

[11] Yahshua- Hebrew name for the Son of the One True Living God, Yahweh; Jesus

become a curse for me long before He created me.

Yahshua hath redeemed us from the curse of the law, being made a curse for us: for it is written, cursed is everyone that hangeth on a tree...[12]

---

[12] Galatians 3:13

The Death Sentence

a sentence ordering someone to be put to death for a capital crime

One of the earliest crises I remember was at the age of three years old. For some reason, it appeared that every time I went into crisis mode so did my younger sister, whose name was Billie Joyce. We were two years apart and so at this time, she was one years old. We were both having fun with my father. He loved to put us on his knees and jump us around. Laughing and giggling from ear to ear, we spent the afternoon enjoying each other in our household full of love. As we jumped up and down on daddy's knees, little did we know that the fate of our lives was about to take a very dark turn. Billie Joyce fell ill, and all laughter ceased. Joy dissipated as her body became lifeless. Then, out of nowhere, the attack overtook me, and my body fell victim to agonizing pain. My parents rushed us both to the hospital. Within minutes, we were both comatosed. The doctors had no answers and were not sure what actions to take to cause our lifeless bodies to respond. We were in the hospital for weeks.

We grew up in a small city back in the 1970's, therefore, the doctors were not educated on the disease of Sickle Cell Anemia. By the grace of Yahweh, they consulted a doctor who came in and suggested that they give us blood. Once the blood entered my veins, I woke up out of that comatosed state and was diagnosed with the disease. However, Billie Joyce was not so fortunate. Although, she came out of the coma, she was still fighting for her life. There was a blood vessel in her head that was not allowing proper flow of blood and oxygen to her brain. The doctors went in to do immediate surgery; yet that blood vessel ruptured causing my dear sister to have a stroke. She never fully recovered. At one years old, not only did she suffer from a severe Sickle Cell crisis, but she left that hospital months later unable to walk or talk. She was paralyzed for the rest of her life.

It was the Christmas season, and in my house, Christmas was a special occasion. We not only celebrated the birth of Yahshua, but we also celebrated my birthday as I was also born on Christmas day. I must say despite of the impact that Sickle Cell Anemia had on my family, my parents made sure that we had all we needed, and I was extremely spoiled. This was a different Christmas for our household though. It was the first Christmas in which the curse of this disease was realized in every member of my family's life. Around that Christmas tree were not only presents, but a wheelchair for Billie Joyce. This was the first Christmas where, we as a family, had to embrace the fact that our sister would never talk or walk again. She took on a new form of language that filled the house with awkward sounds of sadness, but at the same time gratefulness that she survived. As mentioned before, the town I grew up in knew little about Sickle Cell Anemia. During this season, in 1976, the Corsicana Daily Sun newspaper came to interview me. They wanted to know how it was to live with Sickle Cell and how it was to have a birthday on Christmas. As I talked with them, I could not let them leave without telling them one of the most important things I wanted for my birthday, "I wish for my sister, Billie Joyce could walk and talk." I did not know then exactly what Yahweh would do with that wish, but I had faith enough to speak it.

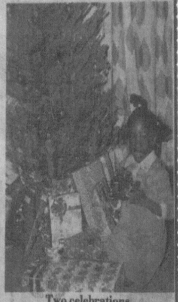

Christi's presents double, but she wants one more

By SYLVIA A. WATERS
Sun Staff Writer

Christmas means two holidays gift wrapped into one for five-year-old Jan Christi Young.

Jan, daughter of Mr. and Mrs. Billy Young, 1218 East 11th Ave., celebrates her birthday Dec. 25 as well as Christmas.

But with all the presents and holiday magic, her birthday wish is an unselfish one.

Jan's being born on Christmas Day took on such a special meaning, her parents gave her the middle name "Christi" taken from Christ. A twin brother died at birth.

"Christmas is quite a holiday around our house," Mrs. Young says.

But Mrs. Young says the family always makes the birthday celebration a special occasion so that it is not overshadowed by all the Christmas festivities.

"Christi is up and wide awake before 7 a.m. We always begin the day by lighting the candles on her cake, singing happy birthday, and opening her gifts," she said.

Christi says she likes having a birthday on Christmas because "You get twice the presents."

She is one of four children and has something she wants Santa to bring each of her sisters and brother.

"I want him to bring Trina (13) a necklace, Andy (11) a watch, and Billie Joyce (4) a teddy bear," she says.

"Oh yes, I want him to bring mother some earrings and daddy a watch," she added.

Christi has the same birthday wish every year before she blows out the candles on her birthday cake.

"You know what I wish for?" she asked. "I wish that my sister, Billie Joyce could walk and talk."

Her sister is a victim of sickle cell anemia and suffers from a stroke.

Her namesake would be proud.

Two celebrations

Five-year-old Jan Christi Young shakes one of the gifts she received for her birthday which will be celebrated on Christmas Day. The best thing about being born on Christmas is getting twice the gifts she says. (Sun Staff Photo by Sylvia A. Waters)

Credits given to Corsicana Daily Sun Newspaper with author and photographer, Sylvia A. Waters.

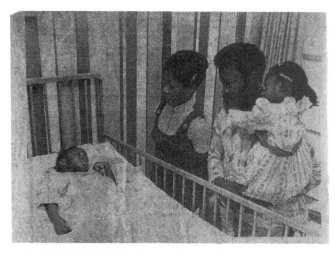

**Credits given to Corsicana Daily Sun
Newspaper with author Jewel Gibson
and photographer, Richard Anderson.**

There was a long journey ahead
for my family and me. Since Billie Joyce
could not care for herself, my precious
mother, quit her job and her pursuit of
a nursing degree and became a full-time
nurse for my sister and me. She did
not want anyone to care for her
children but her. As the crises became
worse and more frequent, the need to
see the doctors became almost a daily

routine. The sad thing about it was that no doctors had answers or could stop the curse. From one doctor to another, they all agreed on one solution, "Mr. and Mrs. Young, the condition of your daughters will never improve, it will only get worse. We can treat them, but we can never cure them. They will never see their adult years."

It was the death sentence given at an early age. The weird thing about it was that neither I, nor my sister, asked for it; nor did we commit any crime that warranted it. It was freely given to us.

I did not know how to take this. As a child who had not even made double digits in age yet, I had a major fight on my hands. I did not know from day to day what to expect with this disease. Each day that I went to school, I was not certain if I would be able to stay a full day. Not only would a pain crisis creep up on me unexpectedly, but the pain of being meddled due to the yellowing of my jaundiced eyes was excruciatingly harsh. It was also tough to see my sister laying on her back every day or sitting in her wheelchair and only being able to move her right arm and her head. Seeing her drove me into prayer daily. I was sorrowful for her and I wanted to do all I could to live the life that she would never have. I made up my mind that I would do all that she would never be able to do for as long as Yahweh allowed me to live. My household became less of a happy place and more of a hostile place. The curse of Sickle Cell Anemia gave birth to more curses within the Young's household. It brought forth the curse of bitterness, the curse of drunkenness, and the curse of physical, emotional, and physiological abuse. My parents felt helpless in that they felt greatly responsible. I remember my father saying "I feel responsible for their condition. I feel I am a bad luck person. I am disturbed that our children would have to suffer because we passed sickle cells to them. I feel guilty."[13] I also recall my mother expressing her grief, "It is like a nightmare learning that Billie Joyce would never walk again. I had no idea that me or my husband had the sickle cell trait. I had no way at that time of knowing."[14]

Sickle Cell Anemia is a very sneaky disease, you could have traits of it and not even know it until it seduces you or your seed with its gripping claws of pain and grief. Everyone should be tested to see if they have it or the trait by taking a simple blood test.

Over the next few years, it became very hard to deal with the devastation of Sickle Cell. It appeared

---

[13] Corsicana Daily Sun -words of my Father.
[14] Corsicana Daily Sun – words of my Mother

that the curse of the disease left from visiting me for awhile and decided to turn all its torment on my sister.

Billie Joyce was getting older. It became more difficult for my mother to pick her up and carry her around the house. She spent most of her days in her special bed or in her wheelchair. Her days became longer, and she was growing tired. I prayed for her daily. There were times that I and my other siblings visited her in the hospital. We knew it was a responsibility of ours to care and love her. She was our dear sister. A few months after her 14th birthday, my parents concluded that it would be best to put my sister in a nursing facility that could help take care of her. We moved from our small town to a larger city where we could be close to her. I was now 16 and preparing to enter the eleventh grade. I was not too happy for the simple fact that I was leaving all my family and friends.

However, I understood the decision that my parents made and that it was in the best interest of Billie Joyce. Every weekend, we went to visit her. She seemed so happy and her smile lit up not only the room, but our hearts, each time we saw her. My parents always diligently checked her to ensure all was well with her and that she was being taken care of as she should. It was hard to leave her, and I can only imagine how my parents felt each time we had to depart and leave her there. My mother had started working part time at the schools in the cafeteria and my dad was focused on expanding his electrician business. It was now only my younger brother and I at home. My oldest brother and sister had gone off to college. I seemed to be during very well in my health. I only had some pain every now and then but no crisis. I no longer had to take medication and it seemed as though I was normal like everyone else. I was overjoyed and ready to take on my last two years of high school. School started, and I became acquainted with this new city and began to develop some friendships.

Christmas rolled around and Billie Joyce was home. It was her first time in the new city and at the new house that we now resided in. She had recently had a birthday and we were all overjoyed that she was home. Time quickly passed, and my parents prepared to take her back to the nursing home. It was a difficult transition, but we all knew that it was the best thing to do at the time.

It was now February 1, 1989. It started out as an ordinary day. My brother and I was preparing to catch the bus for school and my parents were off to work. That day was busy as usual. All seemed to be well. That evening we all made it home and the house was extremely quiet until the phone rang. If I recall correctly, it was my dad who answered the phone. After just a few seconds I heard him scream and for the first time in my life I heard my father cry. At first, we did not know what was going on until he said, "Billie Joyce!" Reality quickly set in that she had passed away. The curse of Sickle Cell Anemia finally gained its justice and the penalty of death took her life at the age of 15.

"For the penalty of sin is death; but the gift of Yahweh is eternal life through Jesus Christ our Lord.[15]

It was a death sentence that each of my family members had to deal with in their own individual way. I truly can only speak about how it impacted me as I only know in part how it impacted them. As for me, I was heartbroken. The doctors were right in their sentencing. My sister was not only robbed of seeing her adult years, but

---

[15] Romans 6:23

she also did not have the opportunity to complete her teenage years. A part of us died with Billie Joyce that day. She was the heartbeat of our family and to see her die so young was almost unbearable.

At the age of 17, in the midst of my grief, all I could think was "I am next." I could not even bear being at her funeral. As I sat on the front seat clutched by the rest of my siblings, I stared at the casket of Billie Joyce and was overwhelmed with grief and terror. All I could think was "I'm next. There is no escaping this sentencing. It's a downward spiral from here. Any hope of me surviving is gone."

Where was Yahweh now? Why did He allow this to happen? Why didn't He answer that one birthday wish? **Why didn't He reverse the curse of the death sentence?"**

Coping with the Pain

physical suffering or discomfort
caused by illness or injury

The Spring of 1989 was filled with dolor emotions. After the passing of Billie Joyce, the Young's household was never the same. For the first time, that I remembered, my mother began to work full time at a local grocery store. My younger brother and I took to our studies and worked hard to focus in a still somewhat new environment. My father was barely seen as he became invisibly clothed in his work, which was mostly out of town. I believe these were the methods that we all used to deal with our grief.

As a junior in High School, it was difficult for me to concentrate at school because I was very different than the average student. First, as the new kid on the block, I had to quickly fit in a huge school population when I was used to a minor crowd who knew everyone. Secondly, not only was I new but my appearance was outside the norm in that everyone wanted to know about the color of my eyes. As a victim of Sickle Cell, I suffered from jaundice. This is a medical condition that causes the yellowing of the skin or of the white of the eyes due to an increased amount of a bodily substance called bilirubin.[16] This is common in Sickle Cell patients because of the excessive breakdown of red blood cells. Some of my peers thought it was cool that my eyes were yellow instead of white. While others joked me into shame. It was often unbearable to deal with the cruelty of their mockery. My self - esteem was very low. It began to affect my ability to focus causing my grades to suffer. There were certain people I intentionally avoided, and I requested to sit in the front of most of my classrooms so I could not see or hear the torment. No one truly understood the pain I was going through with the

---

[16] https://www.medicalnewstoday.com/articles/165749.php

death of my sister, the fear of my own death, and the teasing. I sought comfort but could not find it. I successfully finished my junior and senior years of high school without any crisis or hospital stays. It was as though the storms of Sickle Cell decided to subside from its wrath after the damaged it caused in our household for so many years.

I was at the peak of my health. Regular doctor visits showed that although my hemoglobin level was only half the amount it should be, I was doing very well. The doctors were amazed. I was now married and in my third year of college. I was studying business management as a foundation for law school. The year was 1992 and it was a typical day. I had just finished morning classes and decided to have lunch with a friend. However, I started having some pain in my upper right abdominal area. I was stubbornly insistent in keeping my lunch date. As soon as I reached the office where my friend worked, she immediately looked at me and while looking back at her, I collapsed to the floor. Pain had overwhelmed my entire being. I could barely move. She picked me up and rushed me to the emergency room. The doctors escorted me back and after taking a blood count, they told me that I was having a severe crisis. This attack came out of no where and without warning. It grieved my physical being, weakened my emotions, and tore my dignity. As I laid in that hospital bed succumbing to the many needles, and IVs that were put in my veins, my thoughts went back to the viewing of my sister in her death chamber. The vision of living a normal life quickly fled from my soul as I slowly surrendered to the drugs that were injected into my blood stream to stop the pain. I remembered waking up and screaming. Every inch of me was crying out for relief. The drugs had worn off and I yelled for the nurses to put me out of my misery. I didn't want to be lying in that hospital bed; yet I did not want to be in excruciating pain. I heard the nurses scrambling to get directives from the doctor to inject me with another dose of meds. As they did, relieve came within seconds and I was under its influence, intoxicated, and back in deep slumber. I was not sure what was happening or what the doctors were saying about me. I remember coming in and out of consciousness and seeing my mom's face filled with anguish. No words were spoken as I quickly drifted back into my comfort zone of drugged induced sleep.

A few days passed by and I was finally able to stay awake a few hours to entertain the thought of a meal and brief conversations. My parents paced the floor in search of answers and a way to rescue me from the claws of this disease. My husband was serving in Germany on a military mission and was notified of my dilemma but could not get a leave to come and comfort me due to just returning from leave after our marriage one month ago. I was livid! I wanted answers and I wanted freedom. As a prosperous college student, and newly married bride, I did not have sickness on my agenda. I desired a normal life. Who gave Sickle Cell the right to rob me of what was rightfully mine- the right to live a long and prosperous life, to one day be a mother, and a grandmother, to enjoy retirement, and then die at an old age? Wasn't that the norm for most? Why couldn't it be the norm for me?

Shortly the doctors came in and subtly told me that I would need to have emergency surgery. My liver was damaged, and I had gall stones. They would need to remove my gall bladder.

All major organs are impacted by the abnormal function of tormented sickled cells. The brain, heart, kidney, liver, and lungs are the first to be mutilated. Other organs such as the eyes, gall bladder, and spleen can suffer devastation to the point they no longer function properly due to insufficient blood and oxygen supply.[17]

I was not sure how to take this announcement. I had never had surgery before. Furthermore, the doctors always told me to avoid any kind of surgery due to loss of blood. I prayed and asked Yahweh to cover me and to bring me out of the surgery alive and healthy. The surgery was very quick. They microscopically took the gall bladder out with only three cuts around my stomach area. Although the surgery was simple and successful, the pain was

---

[17] https://www.hopkinsmedicine.org/ healthlibrary/conditions/hematology_and_bl ood_disorders/sickle_celldisease_85,P00101

extreme. They gave me many medications to succumb the pain and to prevent further crisis. I took them for the next ten days as my body healed and recovered leaving signature scars to remind me of my dilemma. Further lab tests showed that my spleen had ruptured and diminished within my internal system. Over the next few weeks I was seeing doctors daily as they continued my treatment.

That winter I flew out to Germany to reunite with my husband. It was an eighteen-hour flight. Although the doctors warned me not to go due to decreases in oxygen in higher altitudes, I went anyway. I took my risk knowing that it was best to live to the fullest degree while I still had breath in my body. The flight was great. I sat toward the front of the plane and watched movies, slept, and enjoyed my adventure. I had never been away from home, my parents, nor outside the

United States! I was proud of the fact that not only did I take a risk, but I took it by myself. The time I spent in Germany was one of the most amazing times of my life. I loved the culture. The weather was blurry cold; but I loved the wintery white snow and the cleanliness of the air. The food was delightful; yet called for an acquired taste. It was the first time I consumed duck, goat, and lamb.

While in Germany, I attended a small church on the base. My husband was a preacher and we often attended after service fellowship dinners with the congregation. I taught the children Bible stories and became very challenged in my own faith. You see I knew of Yahweh from a child and often taught the Bible growing up. I taught what was passed down to me. I read the Bible but had no true relationship with the Bible and I relied heavily on my husband's faith and knowledge. I knew Yahweh loved me and it was by his grace that I was still alive, and that Sickle Cell had not consumed me. I now began to plead for healing as I was often challenged by my husband to believe for it.

After our time in Germany we relocated to a military base in Kansas. We were able to briefly go home to visit with our family and friends prior to relocating. It was so good to see all of them and they were overjoyed that I was doing so well in my health. It had been almost a year since the last crisis.

While in Kansas, we found out that I was pregnant. It was the most wonderful news I could have received. We quickly found a doctor who began to care for me. Things seem to be going well after my first visit. I was then six weeks into the pregnancy. Another six weeks passed by and I was now twelve weeks. I was so excited and had thoughts of the bundle of joy I was carrying.

Then trauma encaged us again. I began to have excruciating pain that would not stop. My belly began to ache as in turmoil. I was rushed to the hospital and they performed a D & C which is a dilation and curettage to cut tissue out of my uterus due to a miscarriage. I was furious as I felt Sickle Cell had robbed me again. Yet through my anguish, I mustered up enough faith to say that I would try again. Two years later, we once again received the news that I was pregnant. The fear and sorrow of what happened in the past diminished and joy and ecstasy filled my world. I knew Yahweh would answer my prayer and give me double for my trouble. I was pregnant with twins and could not wait to tell my parents knowing that they would be overjoyed because they would now experience the excitement of twins in the family since my twin died at birth. This is what my thoughts pronounced to me every day. Yet my husband and I only told our closest friends and decided to wait until I was further along in the pregnancy before telling the family. I was now twelve weeks pregnant. My husband's uncle passed away and he had to travel home to eulogize him. We thought it best for me to stay back and rest in order to maintain the healthy progress of the pregnancy. My husband was not gone a full 24 hours when I started having problems. I began spotting. The doctors placed me on bed rest and told me to wait it out to see if the spotting would stop. In the darkest hour of the night, a painful blow hit my stomach. I could barely move. I felt the flow of blood gushing down. I got up and forced myself to the bathroom. While holding my vaginal area with one hand, I reached to turn the light on with the other. I slowly lifted my bloody hand only to see a glob of fleshly embryo pieces staring back at me. It was a nightmare that I will never forget. I screamed and fell to the floor weeping.

As I sat on the bed in the emergency room waiting for the doctor, I looked at the clock. It was 4:55 am. I tried to reach my husband with no success. The doctors came in with the charts and asked me questions in which I can not recall. All I remember was the visions of my bloody hands and the remains of the dead fetus as though they came alive to mock at me and remind me that the doctors warned me not to try to have children. The doctors continued to tell me. "You do not have enough blood in your body to have a child. Either you would die, or the baby would die, but you both will never survive." This was the death sentence all over again that would forever be my fate. As the doctors left the room, I stayed sitting on that bed numb. All hope was gone. I felt I was robbed from the very thing I wanted most and that was to be a mother. Again, I asked myself, where was Yahweh? Soon a nurse came in and told me I would have to leave the emergency room. There was no need to do a D & C because my body had successfully rejected and ejected the fetuses out of my womb as though it was some foreign substance. How could such havoc be a success?

This was too painful. I could not bear the thought of failing to give my husband kids and my parents grandkids. I could not bear the pain of knowing that I would never have a child to call me "mommy". It was unjust and I felt there was no need to serve a God who could not be touched with my emotions or be kind to my plea for healing and restoration.

I had yet to understand how this test would become a testimony;

nor did I know at the time the great reward that would be reaped from this seed of adversity.

After this I went into months of crisis one right after the other. There were times I went into the hospital demanding drugs that were easily given to me. Two such drugs that I embraced were Demerol and Hydrocodone. At any sign of pain, I called up my doctor and had a prescription filled within moments. You may ask how I was able to pay for all the medical expenses and the supply of pain medications. I had been on Medicaid since I was diagnosed with Sickle Cell Disease. All my medical expenses were paid for plus I received a disability check every month. Now as an adult those checks were sent to me in my name. One of the reasons I want to stress these facts is that Sickle Cell can easily become a mind disease that can drive a person to live a lazy, unproductive, and feeling sorrowful life, if they are not cautions to its crucifying effects.

Many people with Sickle Cell have become addicted to the pain medications. This is mostly due to the fact that over a certain period of time, the body becomes immune to certain prescription drugs. This quickly leads to tolerance which requires higher dosages to be taken to have the medical impact. Physical dependency on the drugs set in when the user's brain changes due to the drug use. The user then becomes reliant on the drug in order to function normally.[18]

This is exactly what happened to me. I was slowly becoming addicted to the "high" the medicines gave me. I wanted to be taken out of my misery and not have to think about the physical and emotional pain that this

_____

[18] https://dictioncenter.com/opiates/demerol/

disease was tormenting me with continuously. I did not want the reality to set in that I, like Billie Joyce, would soon reach my doom. As one who was coping with various forms of pain, I began to fake crisis mode. I knew because of my valid medical history that the doctors would not check my body. They would only ask me if I felt I needed to go into the hospital. My blood count was always at a level that pointed to crisis mode. Therefore, there were times I decided to stay in the hospital because it had now become my comfort zone and my safe place. Then there were times when I just took the supply of drugs given to me in order to use them at my leisure. I felt myself changing. I no longer had a will to do all my sister would never have the opportunity to do. Sickle cell had sucked the drive out of me and I could not see past this point. All I wanted to do was sleep my misery away

and that is exactly what the drugs
helped me do.

The Breaking

to separate (something) into parts or pieces often in a sudden and forceful or violent way

Now at the age of 24, my life lacked buoyancy. Each day was greeted with the caricature mockery of a dispensation of pitiful times that was never ending. I began to embrace the fact that any hope of living a healthy and productive life was doomed. All that surrounded me was the medical permanence that was proven over and over again. Sickle Cell had spoken, and its curse refused to be forsaken.

As I looked back over the last few years of my life, I began to lose control. I was in survival mode and soaked in all that the doctors told me as I let them take my fate into their own hands. I was now actively going to the cancer wards weekly to receive shots of Procrit. Procrit injections were given to chronical ill patients to help them cope with the calamitous effects of long - term diseases such as cancer, HIV, and kidney disease. The medicine is used to increase the red blood cell count and to reduce the need for chemotherapy or blood transfusions.[19] The doctors also had me take daily nasal dosages and many other types of meds. I slowly relinquished my will to fight. My stubbornness to believe that Yahweh would heal me was slowly wrestled away as the doctors eulogized my dreams of living a healthy life. Unbeknownst to me, the medicines were not only reducing my mental state, but they were also internally damaging my nervous system, and my body's ability to cope normally with infections. It was like the enemy seductively forced his will of defeat on me as I ignorantly rested in what was being verbally and medically given to me. Then, all of the sudden, my life shifted in a way I never saw coming.

It all started one morning when I woke up in extreme pain. My legs and

_____

[19] https://www.webmd.com/drugs/2/drug-34/procrit-injection/details

knees were swollen and screamed with agony. Due to my body dripping with sweat, I took my temperature and it was 104 degrees. I never remembered it ever being that high before. My husband was prepared to take me to the emergency room. But I stopped him. This was a Sunday morning and I knew that once I got to that hospital the doctors would keep me there for days, if not weeks. I begged my husband to allow me to go to church. I needed to talk to the Father.

While at church, the congregation went into praise and worship. I sat there on the front row, wiping the sweat away and trying to mask my physical and emotional pain. I desired to stand up and lift my hands and join the crowd in songs of praise. Instead, bitterness set in and I angrily bowed my head before Yahweh and said, "Lord, I want to praise you too. I want to worship you too, but I can't because I am in pain!" Tears rolled down my face and I began to weep in desperation.

I heard Yahweh speak back to me saying, "*I healed you before I laid the foundation of the world. I am waiting for your faith to catch up with what I have already done.*"

I sat up in a state of confusion. I thought "What do you mean… you already healed me? I don't understand?" I heard nothing back. I could not even remember the rest of the service. I just remember going to the hospital afterwards, and as I already knew, I stayed in that hospital for three weeks as they worked to treat the unusually low blood count and lower the infections that resulted in the high fever. Once again, I found myself nursed by the overwhelming calmness that the drugs brought to my mind and body. For me this was the place of peace and tranquility. After a few days, the number of meds were lowered, and I came back to my right mind. I could not wait till visiting hours were over and everyone was forced to leave my room. I yearned to hear Yahweh's voice again. I had so many questions to ask him. I wanted to tell him how I felt and allow him to embrace my fears. Yet, it seemed the more I prayed, the quieter it became. He would not speak to me, at least that is what I thought. The next day, an African American doctor came in. He examined me and began to ask me a few questions that I had never been asked before. He asked me about my eating and drinking habits. He also asked me to tell him all that I knew about Sickle Cell. During this conversation, I had to admit to him that I was not drinking the recommended amount of water for a healthy human being, nor was I consuming the proper amount of fruits and vegetables. My eating habits were poor, and I chose carbonated, sugary drinks over natural water. As far as my knowledge of Sickle Cell, I only knew parts of what I heard the doctors tell me and most of that I barely understood.

As if he took the role of my father, this doctor began to chastise me. He told me that if I wanted to live, then I must immediately change what I put in my body and increase the knowledge of what was going on with my condition. He went on to demand that I ask questions and investigate, if not challenge, the information being spoken over my life. It was crucial that I understood the medications and their side effects. He left me puzzled by his last few statements reassuring me that there was a better way, even if it meant looking at a more naturalistic and spiritual health routine. On the day that I was dismissed from the hospital, this same doctor came to visit me and gave me a prescription for *folic acid*. He told me that this was also an over the counter supplement that I could purchase. It would help my body produce and maintain new red blood cells without the addictive influence. He reminded me of the previous conversations we had, and he wished me well. As I look back now, this doctor was sent by Yahweh to continue the conversation I longed to have with him. **Yahweh comes in many forms. We must be open at all times to discern his voice**.

Once discharged from the hospital, I decided to take on the challenge that was given to me. I purchased a journal that I would use to document my findings of sickle cell and the future conversations that I would have with the doctors.

My husband was now preparing to leave the military after completing the required years of service. We both agreed that we needed a new atmosphere and decided to move to Arlington, Texas. You see, not only was my husband a leader in the military, but he was also a ministerial leader in our church. I did not know how my illness toiled him, but I knew that he needed a break and longed to be ministered to.

It was the year of 1996 and Bishop T.D. Jakes had just opened his new church in Dallas, TX. We were searching desperately for a new church home but was not quite ready to join such a huge congregation. Therefore, we attended Saturday night services. As we settled into our new environment, it seemed as though a new charge to live caused my fears to be swept underneath all the joy and excitement. You see I had listened to Bishop T.D. Jakes for years and I could barely wait to get to his church and hear him say. "Get Ready, Get Ready, Get Ready!!!!" I truly was ready for a change in my life. For some reason my heart soared with expectations of being healed and renewed in my body and my soul. What was ahead of me could have never been imagined. **In order to be healed, I found out that you first must be broken.**

It was a Saturday night and my favorite singing artist was there, *Witness.* They sang a song called, "The *Blood*". It was about the story of how the blood of the lamb was spread over the houses of the Israelites to protect them from the death angel as they prepared to exit their state of slavery. *"It is the blood of the lamb that removes the stain of sin from the heart of man. There is power in the blood that ran down his side.*[20]   This song so ministered to me in that **I needed Yahshua's blood to cover the insufficiency of what my blood could not do. My blood could not**

---

[20] Witness, Album – A Song in the Night, The Blood

protect me from the death sentence over my life, but the blood of Yahshua could.

♪ *"What can wash away my sin? What can make me whole again? Nothing but the blood. Power in Blood. Oh, there is Power in the blood..He was wounded for my transgressions. There is Power.. It's in the Blood..He was bruised for my iniquities..It's in the blood… Wonder working Power..It's all in the blood..There is a fountain filled with blood drawn from Immanuel's vein. It's in the blood. Yes it is..talking about the Blood of Jesus. It's in his blood that I have joy, I can go through because of the blood."*[21] ♪

You see it is no coincidence that Sickle Cell is a blood disease. They say that there is no cure; but the truth of the matter is that *Jesus surely hath borne our griefs and carried our sorrows: yet we did esteem him stricken, smitten of*

---

[21] Witness, Album – A Song in the Night, The Blood

Yahweh, and afflicted. But he (Yahshua) was
wounded for our transgressions, he (Yahshua)
was bruised for our iniquities: the chastisement
of our peace was upon him (Yahshua); and
with his (Yahshua) stripes we are healed!!!![22]

The very fact that healing is a process
was something that I had to learn and
within these verses, you find the
process to healing. You see, deep in my
heart I was still grieving the death of
my sister. Each and every time I was
faced with a crisis or minor health
challenge, I thought about her untimely
death and what the doctors spoke over
my life. I slowly found out that I did
not have to carry that grief because
Yahshua had already borne or carried it
for me. The sorrowful tears I
continuously wept did not have to
continue because Yahshua collected
them for me and He promised to keep
track of all my sorrows and record each

---

[22] Isaiah 53:4-5

one.[23] Therefore, one of the first things I did was take all my grief, sorrow, and tears to the Most High God. In prayer, I bowed before Yahweh and I began to talk to Him about the pain I felt, and how I did not understand why at the age of five years old, He never answered my prayer to heal my sister. I let Yahweh know that I was fearful of my own life and that every night I was taunted by the fear of death. As I poured my tears out to Him, I felt as though some heavy object was being lifted off my entire being. I could not explain it, but I knew something moved. Unbeknownst to me, it was now time for the second stage of healing.

One thing I loved about being at the Potter's House was that Bishop Jakes taught the Word in a way that I could clearly understand it and he

---

[23] Psalms 56:8

challenged what I thought I knew about Yahweh and my responsibilities to Him as His child. Growing up in a traditional church, my knowledge of Yahweh was very limited. I did not know He cared so much about every aspect of our being. As Bishop taught about the afflictions of the children of Israel, one thing stuck out at me and that was that this was a group of people who were chosen by Yahweh and was loved so deeply that their most gruesome crimes did not turn his face or promises from them. **Yahweh is a God of love, grace, and mercy and his hand of forgiveness and restoration is ever so present.** As I listened to the sermons and focused on the mistakes that were made from the first family of Adam and Eve, to this mighty nation who was going into slavery for failure to acknowledge their transgressions toward the one true God, thoughts of my childhood began to flood my head.

I saw myself as a little girl hiding under my neighbor's bed. There all alone, I was shivering and overwhelmed with fear for my mother. Everything within me wished she was there with me and that our circumstances were different. You see I briefly mentioned how the curse of Sickle Cell birthed more curses within our household. The curse of abuse poured its wrath on my mother without failure and its residue greatly impacted me and the lives of my siblings. There were times my drunken father beat my mother so bad that we, as children fled to our neighbors and relatives' houses by foot. We were drenched with fear, sorrow, and grief. It was not until my adult years that I found out from my oldest brother and sister how they were impacted too. Although the physical abuse subsided after the death of my sister, it still impacted all of us in similar ways. One similarity was the failure of experiencing successful marriages. I can only tell my story here as I could never do justice for my siblings. The first five years of my marriage to my husband was nothing short of insanity. Without effort or valid reason, I found justice in faulting the one man I loved of treason. I always put before him the statute, "If you ever hit me, I am leaving you." I did not realize that every time I said that I was creating an atmosphere of war and mistrust. I never thought he would hit me, but it was my defense mechanism to prevent reliving my past. I created a nest of chaos and confusion. There was no room for my king to lay his head in my house, and there was no peace unless I had my way. As I sat under Bishop's ministry, I began to realize my sins and knew that I could never be free from the cage of my childhood unless I faced every ghost that subtly seduced me, and all attached to me.

Yahweh began to deal with my heart. He showed me my iniquities and transgressions. I could no longer hide under the bed of my childhood and make excuses; for the Bible clearly tells us that when we were children, we spoke, understood, and thought like children, but when we become adults, *mature in our understanding,* then we must put away childish things.[24] As the loving Father that He is, Yahweh began to show his mighty hand of discipline in my life. Tears of brokenness began to flow as I cried before Yahweh and surrendered to the fact that in order to be healed, I had to allow him to chasten me and chisel away every attitude, demeanor, fear, and distrust that held me captive. Therefore, for the next few weeks, my husband and I came together and talked about my past pain that attempted to erode my future. I repented to him and asked for his

---

[24] 1 Corinthians 13:11

forgiveness. We prayed for my healing and deliverance. Finally, I was free to love from a pure and untainted heart. **You see Yahweh did not just send his son to die for our sins, but He died for our condition also. The blood of Yahshua covered every injustice that could ever be made against us and because he was wounded, we *were* healed.** That's past tense. **He already provided healing for you before you ever knew you needed a cure.** You must understand, that although healing is provided for you, you must be willing to work for it. That working sometimes calls for brokenness. But **Yahweh is the Master Potter who specializes in breaking His vessels so He can put them back together again.**

My husband and I decided to become members at the Potter's House and the first women's conference was coming up. I was very charged in my spirit to press my way there. I had invited my best friend, Annie Greene, to go with me. Only her and my husband knew about the miscarriages and that I had Sickle Cell Disease.

The first night of the conference was so powerful. The Prophetess that spoke had charged the room with great expectation of what a powerful God could do. I was in great anticipation of Yahweh's presence and I was not disappointed!!! A wave of His glory filled the room leaving no one standing. I was flooded by the Holy Spirit. I could not stop speaking in my heavenly language as I fell to my face in worship. The spirit of laughter came over me as a cloud of unexpected joy filled me. As a drunken woman, I lavishly took it all in. It was just me and Yahweh, everyone else was tuned out and I surrendered to His influence, so much so, that I could not get myself off the floor. My husband came in and carried me to the car as I continued to laugh until 3 am. I drifted into what I thought was a deep sleep. Then something happened that was life changing. Yahweh visited me in my dream. I was laying on a gurney with my eyes glued to the heavens when suddenly, the sky broke open and a huge butcher knife came down towards me. I could not move. A voice from Heaven loudly proclaimed, "*I am going to perform surgery on you. I will take things out of you and put things in you that you will need to do my will.*" I immediately woke up and sat up in my bed. I began to pray to Yahweh for more. I needed more. "Please Lord give me more!!!"

That night I went to service. A woman pastor was the guest speaker. She began to preach about the walls of Jericho.[25] She proclaimed that there were walls that Yahweh wanted broken

---

[25] Joshua 6

down in our lives and that at the shout of faith, they would immediately come down. She explained how there are walls that must be confronted. **You see there are walls in our lives that the enemy has securely built to trap us in. These are walls made up of painful memories, sin, fear, and regret. They prevent us from moving forward and securely keep us from all that Yahweh has for us. At times, we must march around them silently and then command them to break**. If you know the story, the children of Israel were promised that they could have the city of Jericho, but it was barred with a wall. The people were commanded to walk around the wall silently for 6 days. On the seventh day, they would march around the city seven times and the priest would blow their trumpets. At the sound of the trumpet the people would shout, and the wall would come down. Therefore, the pastor had all the ladies count to 7 and then shout. At the shout, there would be massive walls that would come down in our lives. Walls that refused to come down in the past, or at our meager attempts, could not withstand the corporate move of the Holy Spirit. **Through obedience, we must surrender our way of doing things so that Yahweh can have his way.** As I shouted, the Holy Spirit began to rain on me and many other women. I found myself on the floor again as I heard Yahweh clearly remind me, *"I told you I would perform surgery on you and take out all you don't need and put in you all you need to do my will."* Tears of joy washed my soul and my spirit was overwhelmed with ecstasy as I felt fire flow through my entire body. As the service ended, my friend and I escaped the crowd in silence. I knew my life was on a fast track to destiny.

On the third day, Bishop Jakes was scheduled to speak to the ladies.

Before speaking, he had a soloist come to sing. She had a beautiful voice but in the middle of the song, she stopped and said that she had to be obedient and share a recent life experience. She began to tell us how she had just suffered a miscarriage. All of the sudden, my spirit leaped as I heard this woman tell my story. I could not remain seated. I immediately stood to my feet and quietly asked the people sitting by me to excuse me as I passed by them. In my mind, I had to get to a place where I could worship without being disturbed or being a disturbance. I knew that if this woman, who I did not know was telling my story, then Yahweh was about to do something for me.

I quickly found myself at the back of the sanctuary where I fell to my knees and cried out to Yahweh in worship. I thanked Him for bringing me to the church. I thanked Him for touching me and letting me know that He heard me. I heard Bishop take the microphone instructing the ushers to "go and get that woman back there." They came to get me and helped me gain my composure; then they took me to where Bishop was standing. I stood by the soloist. Bishop began to minister to both of us. He laid his hand on my belly and said, "You shall bring forth a child with no problems!" Worship poured out of me and I began to rejoice. I knew I could count on Yahweh. He had answered my prayer, and I still had yet to know all that He was going to do.

Once service was over, my friend went back home to be with her family. I began to read the book that was given to me by a couple on the last day of the conference. It was entitled, "Supernatural Childbirth" by Jackie Mize. My husband and I devoted time every night to read one chapter of the book together. As we began to read, I noticed the book had testimonies of those who had problems giving birth but began to apply the healing power of Yahweh's word to their lives and now had healthy babies with supernatural testimonies. In the back of the book were scriptures and prayers to pray over the baby each trimester. (If you are having problems with childbearing or have suffered a miscarriage, I highly recommend that you read this book. Everyone that I have shared this testimony with and have given this book to now have babies.) Although my husband and I read together nightly, I knew that there was something much deeper that I had to do.

As I read the book, I began to write my own story, you see it was now four months after the conference and I found out that I was once again pregnant!

The doctors began to give me the same sob story of death and doom. But this time I was fully equipped with the weapons of God's word and a promise that was personally given to me. In that book, I began to not only read scriptures about miracles, but I began to write scriptural declarations of my healing from Sickle Cell Anemia.

I listened to the doctors and wrote everything they said down. As I asked questions, I gained knowledge about the disease that I never knew and its impacts on my body. I began to pray for healthy hemoglobin levels to sustain me and the baby growing inside of me. I changed my eating habits to include the necessary vegetables, like broccoli, spinach, and kale, that would build up and reinforce the vitality of my red blood cells. I replaced soda and sugary drinks with a purposeful eight glasses of water daily. I also continued to take Folic Acid daily. At each doctor's appointment I equipped myself with pen and paper to jot down notes and concerns. **As in a war for my promise, I quickly defended my stance that the baby in my womb would not die, but live.** Each time the doctors told me to prepare for the worst, I asked for an alternative for the best. As the doctors expected a miscarriage, I expected and prepared myself for a wholesome nine months of pregnancy. As my husband and I agreed in prayer every night, we brought the growing fetus into prayer also. We laid hands on my belly and began to speak life, health, and strength to the bundle of joy growing inside of me. I also spoke to every red blood cell to live and produce more healthy cells commanding a healthy blood flow to my organs, as well as, to the developing organs of my baby. I reached the twelfth week mark. We rejoiced and praised Yahweh. The doctors suggested to sew my cervix up to prevent a miscarriage. I opted out telling them that the force of the Holy Spirit already did the necessary work and we shall have a healthy baby. At 32 weeks the doctors suggested that I have an amniocentesis done. This is a prenatal test whereby a small needle is inserted into the uterus through the abdomen to withdraw a small amount of amniotic fluid to perform various test on the fetus.[26] The doctors wanted to see if the baby's internal organs were mature enough for her to survive outside the womb. They were suggesting that I consider inducing the labor to have the baby 8 weeks earlier in order to eliminate undue stress to me and the baby. I was at peace with this decision as long as the baby was fine. The Amniocentesis test came back showing the baby's organs were mature and strong. We decided to induce labor at

---

[26] https://www.webmd.com/baby/pregnancy-amniocentesis#1

36 weeks. I was so excited in that in 4 weeks I would have my bundle of joy in my arms. Without any blood transfusions, and with no epidural or medications, I gave birth to a healthy baby girl. Yahweh showed himself mighty in that I did not even know I was in labor. A few hours after receiving the medicine to induce the labor, I told the nurses I needed to go to the bathroom. I thought that I needed to have a bowel movement. The nurse said she wanted to check me first and then she would let me go. Upon checking me she almost screamed with concern for me. She said, "You are fully dilated, and the baby's head is coming out!!! You don't have pain???" I softly said, "No ma'am, what should we do now???." Panic hit the room as my husband released my hand to check out the scene and the nurses yelled for the doctor. He came in and with three pushes, Keturah

Ebony Green was born on September 5, 1997.

Miscarriage no longer had a hold on me, and the curse was broken off my life!

The Bible tells us that *the Kingdom of Heaven suffereth violence, and the violent take it by force.*[27]

Looking back at all these events helped me clearly see that I had to be broken first if I was to break the curse off my life and successfully give birth to another generation. I grew up with a "feel sorry for myself syndrome." I had to learn how to purposely break this off my life and with the guidance of Yahweh's Holy Spirit I was able to successfully embrace levels of breakthroughs in my life through faith and obedience.

---

[27] Matthew 11:12

One such breaking was when I had to decide what I truly wanted in life. Did I want to continue to be a victim or a victor? **Of course, everyone will quickly choose victory over victimization. Yet everyone is not willing to give up the crutches and comfort of being the victim.**

As mentioned in an earlier chapter I was on Medicaid and receiving disability checks each month. I did not have to work if I did not want to. But now I was no longer a victim of sickle cell. At the age of 25, I had not had a crisis or been in the hospital. As a new mom, I wanted to have a vibrant life and blaze a trail for my daughter that she would be proud of. I decided to open a daycare in my home so I could bring money in and at the same time be a stay at home mom helping my husband give her the life we both desired her to have. Because I was working full time, I had to call and report my income. As a result, I received a letter from Social Security informing me that I would no longer receive disability checks while making this income and that I owed the government $1200 due to overpayment from the months I earned income while receiving the checks. I was not thrilled over this, but I decided I wanted to live independent of any disability. Therefore, I paid the money back and received no more checks after that time. Once my daughter turned two years old, I went to work full time for Corporate America in the Financial industry. I have been in management there for over twenty years now.

Prior to my pregnancy, I decided to take myself off all the medications that the doctors had me on. I remembered what the doctor in Kansas told me and I decided to walk out in faith. Either Yahweh would heal me of the devastating effects of Sickle Cell, or I would forever be its victim.

I began to replace the medications with natural foods that carried the things my body needed. I began to purchase vitamins and supplements that I still take today. Vitamin B6 and B12, along with Folic Acid helped me maintain healthy red blood cells. I started making daily drinks with spinach, kale, blueberries and apples that I drink. By during these things, I have not had to take any medications and have not had a crisis. My food became my medication.

Once again, I stress that I am not a physician and I am not advising you to stop taking your medications. I am sharing my testimony to encourage you to seek God for healing and put work behind your faith that will bring about positive change to your situation.

With the help of Yahweh, I walk in healing and no longer a victim of the terror of Sickle Cell Anemia. **The curse has been broken off my life and the death sentence annulled!!!!!**

In 2001, I unexpectedly became pregnant with my second daughter and gave natural birth to healthy Chelsea Renee' Green on June 3, 2002.

Only Yahweh could work such a miracle!!!!

Destined

*Of a person's future developing
as though according to some
divine plan*

According to the Bible we were all on a plan, under a curse, doomed for destruction. We went along with the arrangement already set for us. Due to being born in this sinful world, we were destined to partake of a death sentence that Satan had bargained for. He made a bet with our creator God that we would follow hard after the ways of the world and forsake that inner voice within us that said that we could truly *have life and live more abundantly*.

For the most part, we wholeheartedly ignored that voice and did every wicked thing that our passions or evil thoughts led us into. But because of the rich grace of our God and his love for us, he intervened. He gave us back our lives again, snatching them from the grips of the enemy and his imprisonment. He set us free from the penalty of death by becoming the prisoner himself.

Through the sacrificial death of His son, Yahshua- Jesus, the Christ, our heavenly father redeemed us and BROKE THE CURSE OF THE DEATH SENTENCE off our lives.[28]

Although, I write this book to encourage those who are suffering from the devastating effects of incurable diseases, namely Sickle Cell Anemia, I want you to know that there is a much greater disease. The disease of Sin has so wrecked humanity and put every single human being in a vulnerable state that Yahweh never intended us to be in. The bible says that we have all sinned and come short of the glory of the Lord and that the wages of sin, or what we have to pay because of the sins we committed, is nothing short of death.[29] Our sins have separated us from the one who created us and it was our sins that forfeited our

---

[28] Ephesians 2:1-4
[29] Romans 3:23; 6:23

rights to the inheritance that he has for us. No matter how much our heavenly father wants to reconcile us, he can not even hear our cries of desperation until we acknowledge that He is Lord of Lords, and our innocent savior. It is in him that we live, move, and have our very being. But before we can be released from our imprisonments, we must embrace the truth that He died to set us free.

The bible says that *He so loved the world, that He gave the life of his son, so that if we just believe in him, then we should not perish but have eternal life.*[30] This is what I call *The Great Exchange.* Yahshua came and exchanged our misery for his peace. We no longer have to carry the burdens of sin on our lives or even within our bodies. It is by the beating that He took that we can, not only have life after this life is over, but we can

---

[30] John 3:16

embrace the peace of Yahweh in this life and see His miraculous works in our minds, bodies, and souls. Today, if you are not saved, if you have not acknowledged Yahshua – Jesus, the Christ, as your personal Lord and Savior, as the one who has come to break the death sentence off your life, please say this simple prayer of salvation with me:

Heavenly Father, it is in your son's name, Yahshua, Jesus Christ, that I come before you. I receive the sacrifice that he made for me in dying on the cross, in my stead, for all of my sins. It was his blood that was shed that washes me from all of my iniquities. Lord, I confess with my mouth that you are Lord and that you died and was raised from the dead so that I may have eternal life. I thank you and I now embrace the new life of salvation that you have given to me. Amen!

Amen, welcome my brother, my sister to your new life!!!

Rise Up and Walk

*the act of moving from a lower
position to a higher one*

There is a story in the Bible about a man who was lame from birth. The Bible clearly lays out the fact that this man's ankle bones and feet were weak, which caused him not to be able to walk. He grew up depending on others to carry him wherever he needed to go. Now, as a grown man, he became comfortable with others helping him, and underscoring his incapacity. He found the perfect place where he could rely on others to provide for his every need, even the need to be complacent, allowing his incapability to become his greatest asset. You may ask, what place could that be? Well, the Bible states that it was at the gate of the city's temple. **Could it be that our faith, when unchallenged, entitle our handicaps? Could it be that the very places that should strengthen the areas within our lives that are**

functioning, are the very places that put our inabilities on display?

I want to take a moment to address those who make up the support groups for those with Sickle Cell or other defiant diseases. As a person who grew up suffering from Sickle Cell Disease, I can tell you that my family, church, and community were very important assets that challenged me to either move beyond my frailty or linger in it. Please take into consideration that it was only the man's ankle bones and his feet that were crippled. But everything else was working fine for him. Nothing was wrong with his mind, his hands, nor his mouth. Even his arms, knees, and elbows were strong and worked fine. Yet, when reading the story in Acts chapter 3, we see that after being carried everywhere he needed to go, this nameless man laid at the temple gate every day begging for his means to live. No one challenged him to use what he had. As I read the story, I can't help but ask why didn't his family, friends, and even physicians make provisions for him to strengthen and use those things that remained? In other words, why wasn't a wheelchair created for him or even a walker or canes provided? I am sure there were others that were also lame in the feet; but yet found creative ways to make things happen. Why didn't someone challenge this man to find a skill that he could perfect and eventually get paid for as a productive member of his society? Could it be that those who made up the support group for this man be faulted for him not only being entirely lame, but also nameless? When a person suffers from a dire disease, such as cancer, sickle cell, or epilepsy, just to name a few, they can suffer from emotional anxiety, depression, suicidal thoughts, and low self-esteem that makes them feel like a victim instead of a person. The disease names them to the degree that they have no identity. This is what happened with this man. He laid there at the gate of the temple nameless with his hand outstretched for others to provide for him. The worst thing you can do for your family member, friend, or neighbor that suffers from a disease that disables them in some form, shape or fashion, is to allow them to totally depend on you for their needs. In some way, you must challenge them to think outside their situation, use what they have and strengthen it, and find a way to be productive. Then, and only then, will they feel like they have something to give and that they are important. Despite of their illness, they are valuable and must come to embrace the fact that they are still alive because of purpose!

When we continue to read in Acts 3, we see that the man's situation did not change until he was challenged. It was the wisdom of Peter and John that caused this lame man to rise above his lameness and find his identity. They refused to give him a handout and instead gave him a hand up. They prayed for him and then provoked him to act on his faith. **If you have a love one who is suffering from an incurable disease, you must not only pray for them and with them, but you must provoke them to put their faith to work.** The bible tells us that faith without works is dead being alone.[31] Acts tells us that as Peter and John approached the man, they did not acknowledge his request for money, but they told him, "*We have no money for you, but in the name of Jesus Christ of Nazareth, rise up and walk.*[32] With that being said, they grabbed him by something that was working for him.

---

[31] James 2:26
[32] Acts 3:6

They grabbed him by his right hand, lifting him up, and the Bible says that immediately his feet and ankle bones gained the strength he needed to not only walk, but leap into the temple!!!!.

Remember my earlier testimony that started with a challenge? I had to decide whether to give up a Social Security Disability check each month in exchange for wholeness. I decided that I did not want to be lame anymore, it was because of the faith that was instilled in me that I believed that I no longer had to be lame but that I could indeed leap. Now I am not telling you to do all the things that I did. But for me, it was a matter of life or death to stop taking all the medications and walk in the faith of God's word that said, *"I shall not die, but live, and declare the work of the Lord." As I write this book,* I travel and speak to crowds of people encouraging them to believe on the one true God and challenging them to identify and live out their purpose. I minister to those that suffer from the same affliction that use to encage me and I let them know that they too, no longer have to be a victim but with faith, backed up with works, they too can be a victor!!

As far as that nameless lame man, the Bible tells us that all that knew him in his lameness now wondered in amazement of his empowerment. As he leaped, he drew crowds that wanted to hear about the miracle that took place in his life. He became a drawing agent for those that had no hope. For those who suffer, could it be that there are people waiting for you to step out on faith and strengthen the things that remain working for you? For those that support the ones suffering, could your love one, neighbor, or church member be waiting on you to challenge them to embrace the abilities that God has given to them in order to be productive and feel like they have something to offer to the environment that they partake in on a daily basis? **It is in the ability to rise above the victim mentality, does one find their true identity.**

True identity is not what the doctors or your situation says about you. True identity is what God said about you before you were even formed in your mother's womb. Through prayer and reading the Word of God, your true identity can be revealed to you and it shall speak louder than any circumstance, disease, or trouble that you are facing. I gave you my testimony and the strategies I took to get me where I am today. Through prayer and supplication, God will give you your own testimony and the strategy that you need to take to get you there. Rise up and walk! Rise up from your lameness and began to leap in all that God has said about you and all that He says you can have! As you leap, watch anxiety, depression, emotional distress, and low self-esteem disappear as others wonder in amazement of your new abilities.

As you prepare to rise, start with some practical methods to help you gain your momentum. First, educate yourself on the disease. Whether you are the caregiver, part of the support system, or the actual patient, you must find ways to educate yourself on the disease. In our world today, knowledge is no longer hidden. In my lifetime, there were times I had to rely on the doctors to tell me information that they did not want to give to me but was certainly my right to have. That is not the case today. Just by googling Sickle Cell, you can find out all you need to know about the disease. You can also google common factors, and underlying causes of the disease, and information about the medications being prescribed to you and their side effects. You can google natural remedies that you can take instead of the medicines being prescribed and take that information to the doctor so you both can work together on a regimen that is right for you. Being educated, not only gives you knowledge about what you are facing, but it gives you the upper hand and a say so on how you prefer to be treated. Ask questions and challenge anything you feel uncomfortable about and request options as you deem necessary.

Once you are educated, speak life to your body and write your own story. Read stories in the Bible about healing, such as the story of the lame man. Put yourself in those stories and see yourself healed. Find every scripture in the Bible that speaks life and declare them over yourself. Write out your declarations and post them where you can see them daily and take time to declare them over your life. Command your body to line up with what you read and speak. **Remember, healing starts with your mind. You must see yourself healed before the healing begins to physically manifest**. Next, seek God for His promise to you. Don't be so quick to agree with what others say about you and your situation. Sometimes you must even abandon your own mind about yourself. Seek God for what He is saying about you. Remember He wrote your ending before your beginning. He already has a solution for you and once you uncover it, you will become it. Go to war for your promise. No one can do this for you. You must pray and read God's word for yourself until you hear Him clearly speak to you about what He has promised you. Then speak that promise into every area that is opposite to it until those areas line up with what you are decreeing.

Changing what you put in your body is another effective way of rising above the illness. If you research the illness that you suffer from, then you will soon discover various foods and supplements that can help you heal and overcome the devastating effects of the disease. Because Sickle Cell is a blood disease that attacks the normalcy of red blood cells, I found out that it is necessary to eat foods that would reduce anemia and increase the production and longevity of hemoglobin for red blood cells. Supplements such as folic acid, B12, and iron were things I discussed with my doctor. I also discussed my willingness to take these supplements, along with foods such as kale, spinach, broccoli, black beans, kiwi, pomegranate, and avocados to increase my red blood cell production. I agreed to come off sodas and sugary drinks and increase my intake of water, along with fresh green smoothies in exchange of the doctors monitoring me as I took myself off all the medications they put me on. My body slowly responded to my new regimen. Once my body adapted to the healthy diet, then it supernaturally began to yield to healing instead of devastation. As a result of my education and knowledge, I prevailed in finding a way to avoid the negative impacts of medications that only placed a band-aid on the symptoms but never healed me of the disease. **God is no respecter of person, if you put the work behind your faith, God will also give you the means to prevail!**

Live on Purpose

*the reason for which something
is created or for which
something exists*

Now that you have the mindset to walk in healing, what will you do once the curse of sickness and disease is broken off of you? Earlier, I mentioned how the lame man became an inspiration to others as they looked at him leaping and walking. I am a true believer that healing comes for the sole reason of giving you the power and authority to walk out the purpose and plan that God has for your life. The bible tells us that there shall be no more curse; but the throne of God and of the lamb shall be in the place of healing and restoration. In that place all of his servants shall serve him.[33] Of course this verse speaks of the time when God will restore this evil world with his presence and there will be no more death, disease, or sickness. It will be a time when our relationship with God will be restored as He originally intended, and all sin will be destroyed.

---

[33] Revelation 22:3

Yet, I want to encourage you that you can partake in a portion of this joy now. The question I have for you is **Why should God answer your prayer for healing? What will you do once you are healed?** Began to seek God now for greater clarity on why He put you in the earth realm. Furthermore, I want to challenge you to ask God what He had in mind for you when He allowed you to be afflicted with the disease or illness you are currently suffering with. The Bible tells us that all things work together for the good to those that love God and who are the called according to *purpose*.[34] There's that word Purpose again. If you love the Lord, and even if you don't know him that well, please know that HE LOVES YOU and has good intentions towards you. His plans and purpose for you are plans of peace, and not of evil to give you an expected end- a purpose

---

[34] Romans 8:28

for his glory.[35] Having the illness that you or your loved one suffers from is not an indication of God being angry at you or punishing you for something you did. Could it be that He has chosen you so that He can do a miracle through you so that many people that know you will be strengthened in their faith later when they witness you overcome?

There is a story in the bible that proves this. It is about a man who was blind from birth. People asked Jesus, "Who did sin, this man, or his parents, that he was born blind?" Jesus told them that no one sinned; the man was born blind so that God's work of healing could be manifested through him.[36] But let me drive it home even more by telling you some things God has done for me through Sickle Cell. I recall lying in the hospital bed in

---

[35] Jeremiah 29:11
[36] John 9:1-3

Junction City, Kansas. They brought in a young lady who became my roommate. She was suffering from congestive heart failure. She wanted to give up on life due to the bad news the doctors had given to her about her heart condition. While lying in that hospital, I sat up and began to minister to her. I spoke life to her situation and prayed for her. Her whole demeanor changed, and she began to talk positively about her future. She believed God for healing. Two days later, test results came back saying her heart condition had improved drastically to where no surgical procedure would need to be done and with medication, the condition of her heart would go back to normal. She was so overjoyed and left the hospital praising God. She visited me during the remaining week until I was released. But my point is what if I was not in the hospital during that time? I saw purpose in my affliction to help someone else overcome theirs. Another incident I remember is being a trainer at a financial company. I trained hundreds of employees weekly. One day, as I released my class, I noticed a young man who was still siting at the back of the class once everyone cleared the room. His head was cradled in his arms on the desk. I walked to where he was and asked if he was okay. With tears in his eyes, he explained to me that his wife had called informing him that she had just miscarried their first baby. I ministered to him and asked him to see me the next day. I went home and purchased the book *Supernatural Childbirth*. Enclosed I put a letter that I wrote to him and his wife about my testimony of having several miscarriages and now a mother of a healthy baby girl. I wrote my contact information in the book. The next day I gave him the book and asked him to promise me that he and his wife would read it. He promised. I never saw him again but a year later, I went to my mailbox and found a surprise. It was a package from an unknown sender. I opened it up and pulled the book out. Inside was a letter from the gentleman and his wife and a picture of their newborn baby! I was so overjoyed and praised God for allowing me to help this family. You see I could not have helped them if I would not have suffered a miscarriage myself. **Your pain is tied to purpose. Your ability to overcome is tied to someone else being able to overcome as well**. Seek God for purpose so that as you began to walk in that purpose, healing will overtake you.

As I write this book, I minister to many people with various forms of Sickle Cell. I go to the hospitals to encourage and pray for them. I even host support groups in my city. My declaration is "Devil you messed with the wrong one!!!" If he knew that I would be ministering to many and helping them overcome sickness and disease, he would have never terrorized my home. I am believing with you that the same God that has given me a strategy to overcome the devastating effects of Sickle Cell Disease will touch your mind and body and give you a strategy of success that when you put it into effect, many will be encouraged and touched by your life and testimony. There is purpose in you living. If it wasn't, you would have been taken out a long time ago by your dilemma.

Declarations and Prayers

When praying to God about healing for my body and overcoming the devastating effects of Sickle Cell Anemia, I spoke the following declarations over my life daily and prayed these prayers. I hope you find that they work for you also. Feel free to write your own declarations and prayers that fit your situation. **Then believe in your heart that what you ask for is already yours and began to walk in the reality of it**. It is very important that you also do the work. Change your eating habits and your thought process. Work with your doctor to come up with the best regimen for you. Last, but most importantly, Live on Purpose!!!!

Philippians 4:6-7 Be careful for nothing; but in everything by prayer and supplication with thanksgiving let your requests be made known unto God.

General Prayer for Healing

Gen. 1:27 So God created man in his own image, in the image of God created he him; male and female created he them.

Romans 8:21-23 - Because the creature itself also shall be delivered from the bondage of corruption into the glorious liberty of the children of God. For we know that the whole creation groaneth and travaileth in pain together until now. And not only they, but ourselves also, which have the first fruits of the Spirit, even we ourselves groan within ourselves, waiting for the adoption, to wit, the redemption of our body.

Galatians 3:13 - Christ hath redeemed us from the curse of the law, being made a curse for us: for it is written, cursed is everyone that hangeth on a tree:

Psalms 118:17 - I shall not die, but live, and declare the works of the Lord.

God when you created man, you said that he was "good". You did not create us with disease, disorders, or abnormalities. You created us healthy, strong, and perfect like you. But because of sin, the whole earth groans.

Lord, as your child who has given her life to you, I have been redeemed from the curse of the law. By your blood you redeemed me when you died for me. Therefore, Lord, I decree that by your stripes I am healed. So, I come against this illness and I will walk in healing. I command my body to line up with your word. I shall not die but Live and declare the works of the Lord. In Jesus' name, Amen.

Prayer Specifically for Sickle Cell Symptoms

Isaiah 53:5 - But he was wounded for our transgressions, he was bruised for our iniquities: the chastisement of our peace was upon him; and with his stripes we are healed.

Lord, I acknowledge that you suffered for all of my bodily infirmities, weaknesses, and diseases. Therefore, I accept that you have provided healing for me in all areas when you took those stripes on your back. As a result, I not only proclaim healing, but I now walk in total and complete healing of my body.

Sickle Cell Anemia no longer has a hold on me. I declare and decree that all my red blood cells are healthy, normal, and whole. I speak to my red blood cells to be round shaped, narrow, and not sickled shaped. Red blood cells, you shall have a normal life cycle of about 110-120 days, and you shall be healthy and strong. My red blood cell count shall be normal at 4.2 to 5.4 million red blood cells per microliter (normal for adult female).

I rebuke the process of hemolysis and I speak an increase in hemoglobin in my red blood cells so that they circulate and function properly to carry oxygen to all my bodily organs. My hemoglobin level shall be normal at 12-16 grams per deciliter of whole blood. The CBC test shall reflect this normalcy.

In Jesus name, and by the stripes you took for me, I thank you now that anemia has no place in my physical body.

Brain, nervous system, kidney, liver, spleen be healed in Jesus name!

As my body lines up to the healing that Jesus gave to me, Jaundice shall be eliminated, and all tests shall reflect normalcy. In Jesus' name. Amen.

Additional Prayers for Forgiveness and Healing

Psalms 103:2-4 - Bless the LORD, O my soul, and forget not all his benefits: Who forgiveth all thine iniquities; who healeth all thy diseases; Who redeemeth thy life from destruction; who crowneth thee with lovingkindness and tender mercies;

Lord, I thank you for forgiving me of all of my sins and iniquities and for healing me of all my diseases. You are my Jehovah Rophe, the God that healeth me. Thank you for redeeming my life from the curse of disease and destruction and giving me long life because of your love, kindness and mercy towards me.

Psalms 91:16 - With long life will I satisfy him and shew him my salvation.

Lord, because of your promise to me, I shall walk in healing and have long life upon the earth and because of my healing, many others shall also walk in their healing.

My Personal Declaration

I will walk in complete physical healing. As a result of my healing, I will lay hands on the sick and they shall recover. There is healing in my hands and I will bring healing to men and women who are hurting. Because of how God will use me and the pain he allowed me to endure, many will come to understand the purpose for their lives and walk in it.

Letter from the Author

Beloved, I wish above all things that thou mayest prosper and be in health, even as thy soul prospereth.

3 John 2

As you have read the pages of this book, my prayer for you is that the words have resonated deeply within your spirit. I pray that something that I have shared has become food for your soul in such a way that you find faith, hope, and the healing that you so long for.

Recently God gave me a meaning for the world's term of DEJA VU. Worldly, the term means "already seen. When Deja Vu occurs, it sparks our memory of a place, event, or person we may have already encountered. Well in the spirit, God gives us **Déjà vu** moments. His definition to me is as follows: **Divine Eternal Journeys Aspired by Victorious Utterances**. You must know that God desires the best for you. He has set up a future to prosper you in every area of your life. Throughout your journey, there will be times when you will receive glimpses of what is to come. This is to stir your faith and to cause you to desire more. Keep walking. Because when life gets tough, and the storm clouds roll in, if you keep walking, you will soon see the rainbow. When you arrive to your destination, the places, the events, the healing, the purpose that God has for you, it will seem as though "I already been here before." You have because your destiny was planned out before you were even born. This is why God told me *"I healed you before I laid the foundations of the world. I am waiting for your faith to catch up with what I already done*!"

God has done the work. You must walk the journey that he has laid before you out. This journey is **Divine** because it is of Him. No matter what it looks like, no matter how hard it may be, know that it is **a journey** God has laid out for you. It is an **Eternal Journey** that started before your momma gave birth to you. It initiated in the presence of the most holy God and it will continue on way after you leave this earth. Your journey is **Aspired**. That means it is directed towards achieving greatness. The reason why is because God is directing it and if you listen closely, the Holy Spirit whispers **Utterances** to you that are **Victorious**. By your faith, you shall have all that you desire. Keep believing. Keep walking and partner with the Father on this journey. Your journey! Your DÉJÀ VU!

Blessings to you always,

Jan Christi Green

To book Jan Christie Green for speaking engagements or for questions about other products or services, please reach out to:

jchristi Global Connections at

Website:

www.jchristiglobal.com

or

Email:

info@jchristiglobal.com

Or call us at: 682.593.2750

We look forward to serving you.

Made in the USA
Lexington, KY
20 December 2019